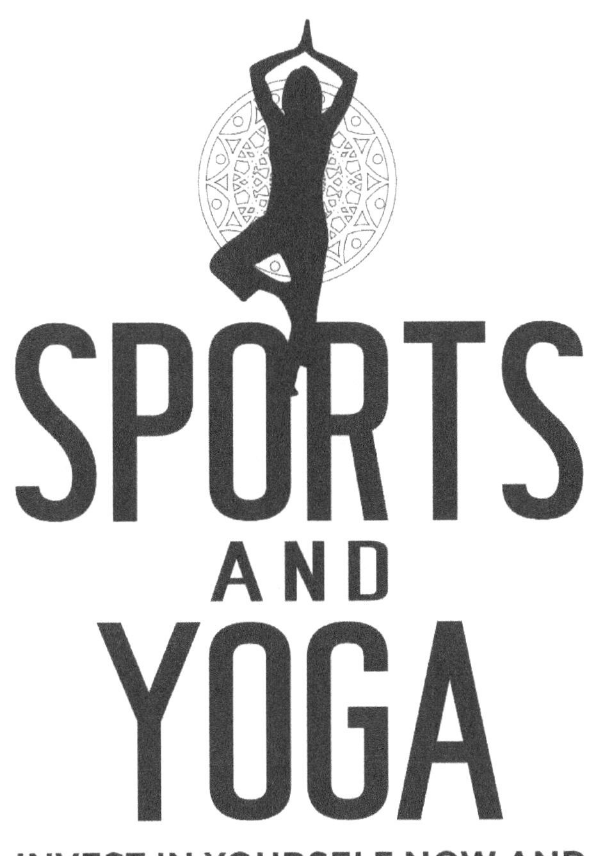

SPORTS AND YOGA

INVEST IN YOURSELF NOW AND YOU WILL THANK YOURSELF LATER

GAV KAY

CONTENTS

INTRODUCTION

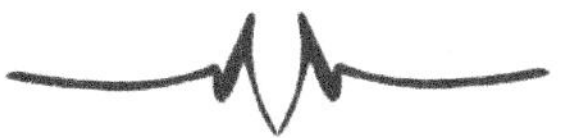

Almost every athlete, professional or not, has had to deal with a sporting injury more than once during the course of their life. This is why many countries and international sporting organizations have adopted this progressive trading technique - Yoga. Yoga has been proven many times to be both preventive and therapeutic. It has positive physical and mental effects on those that practice it, which is why it has been incorporated in the training process of many athletes.

Yoga is distinct and beneficial for every sport; it is also the perfect combination for other forms of exercise. Yoga helps the body function effectively and prevents sporting injuries that may arise from immobility, inflexibility, or other major causes of sporting injuries or muscle tightness. The postures taken help to coordinate breathing and empower all other parts of the body (the muscles, neck, hips, back, shoulder, ankles, and hands). It can also control any imbalance in the development of muscles. All these benefits - stronger body parts, proper development of muscles, coordinated breathing help to prevent sporting injuries and help the injured recover in due time.

There has been a rise in the amount of sporting injuries that require surgeries because of the training method that is focused on increasing muscle mass and strength without flexibility. These injuries would continue to be on the rise if yoga isn't implemented in sports training. Adding yoga to strength training would go a long way in minimizing sporting injuries. What yoga does for the athlete is, it enhances their flexibility which in turn affects their muscles and tissues positively. Also, it gives balance and poise which enable the athlete bounce back from any form of imbalance they might experience during the sporting activity. This is usually an experience for the athlete because they have so much control of their body; they can maximize their body parts and also have an injury-free journey for a long time. For those recovering from injuries, yoga frees the muscles and works to break down scar tissues from old injuries. It is almost impossible for the athlete who has incorporated yoga into their training to experience tightness in the muscles as a result of old age, as most athletes do.

Statistics show a large number of sporting injuries recorded each year for both the young and old. One way to not be part of this large number is to consciously work on your posture, range of motion, balance and flexibility, and yoga helps you with this. With the steady growth of these numbers, it is important that every athlete starts this journey to experiencing an enhanced sporting life both physically and mentally. Yoga and sports are vital aspects of your life and this book is geared towards helping you understand the benefits of yoga in your sporting life and also show you how to fully incorporate yoga into your life enough to get you to realize all its benefits (preventive and therapeutic).

CHAPTER ONE

SPORTS AND YOGA

Yoga is a meditative discipline that has been practiced in the ancient time for flexibility to the spine, the joints, and to strengthen the internal muscles of the person practicing yoga. For some classes of people, yoga was basically to improve their concentration level and create an intense connection between the mind and the body through its meditative practices. For some, it is important for relieving stomach issues and managing body fat to improve their self-esteem and boost their confidence as a result of the physical effect it has on body weight.

However, the benefits of yoga are endless and whatever it is used for, the results have shown positive over the years even in contemporary times. And most especially, as it concerns this book, we would be exploring the implications of yoga on athletes and different sports in this chapter.

To properly understand the relationship between sports and yoga, it is important to first understand the requirements for sporting activities and whether a relationship can exist between the two or not. Actually, the type of sport does not matter whether it is soccer, football, tennis, surfing, swimming, volleyball, or running, they all tend to have the same requirements to ensure good performance, and because of this reason, we would be doing a general check on all sporting events and yoga.

Good performance in sport demands time, energy, and committed practices to build flexibility, stamina, and speed in performance. Aside from that, to perform efficiently, the athlete needs to be fully focused in the moment and confident to perform the task without any slack on any of the grounds I have mentioned especially because of bashfulness. For emphasis, sporting activities demand deep focus, living in the moment with all the distractions and anxiety coming from the crowd and fellow players, with all their booing and cheering. Thus, if a player were to be bashful and lacked stamina, he would constantly fail to make a good pass or score a goal and even when he does, the skillfulness will be missing.

Having seen what it would take, the next step would be exploring the benefits of yoga to see if it could serve any purpose for sporting skills, if it could enhance flexibility, stamina, concentration level, speed and reduce anxiety and timidity as an athlete would require.

Does it really serve a purpose?

Study and practice have shown that yoga practices are directed to controlling breath movements which are later arsenals for improving concentration and mental focus on just anything. The asanas are key here; they help to develop easy mind-controlling and mind concentrating which can be very helpful for sports. The asanas can be beneficial in training the body to develop strong stamina from continuing with its meditative postures on a routine. This is because practices of asanas would have the practitioner focus their mind for the stipulated time of the exercise and what this does in return to the practitioner is help them develop strength in their body and ability to concentrate and focus on their mind.

More than this, the asanas affect the functionality of the body's internal organs in positive ways. Some studies say that they tone the muscles of the body, improve the functionality of the heart and the immune system, stimulate the processes of the circulatory system, enhance weight loss, and alleviate body inflammations. With all these benefits, yoga has got to be very crucial for imminent performance as an athlete because like we have seen it does not only ensure that the mind is focused, but that the body is too. More than just the joints and bones, it benefits the internal organs.

Now, I believe that when we think of yoga, the Asians come to mind, especially the Chinese and the Japanese. It is obviously so because the origin dates back to them and that is why I think it is important that we see the connection of emotions and physical health like the Chinese would see it. They believe that emotions have a specific attraction to certain organs in the body; they believe that fear can harm the kidney and the bladder, that worry anxiety and stress can deteriorate the functionality of the spleen and the stomach, that excess joy can cause injuries to the heart., They believe that grief and depression can hurt the lungs and anger, the gall bladder. They say that sadness makes the brain perform poorly.

I have shared that with you not just because of its credibility, at least for the fact that it is coming from the original owners of yoga practices, but to help you see the importance of yoga in those beliefs.

Yoga moves are in fact targeted to ensure an equilibrium between the feelings the body (internally and externally).

For example, studies show that practicing downward facing dog yoga will stretch the spine, hamstrings, feet, Achilles tendons, and also decrease depressive emotions and reduce anxiety. Cat-cow which will be mentioned later in this book also has been useful for reducing fearful emotions. Worry also is treated with the supine twist yoga that also transcends that to taking care of backaches.

This is why a combination of athletic training and yoga would mean a great performance for any sportsperson and in any sports. The relationship between sports and yoga is simply that it enhances better athletic abilities. By helping them loosen their tight muscle to improve flexibility in tackling and racing, recovering quickly from sports injuries and most of the time, yoga prevents the injuries, nourishes and revitalizes their cells, develops the function of the brain responsible for controlling how the body works in motion, improves muscle coordination and posture balancing important for easy mobility during sporting. It also releases the tensions locked in their body and mind and in the end free their body and mind from the tension and the reasons why they were all tensed up.

I believe that as we progress, we would see more benefits, and how they relate to sporting activities, how it manages to provide them with grace and maximal flexibility and mobility.

CHAPTER TWO

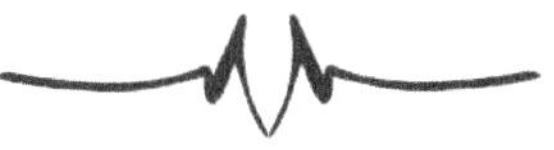

INJURY

According to studies, the most common reason for sports-related injuries is when athletes overuse or abuse their bodies. You can say they incur injuries when they disconnect from their body and take less care of it, most times by overstressing their body and relaxing less than they should.

So, it's easy to propose that the best preventive measure to adopt would be becoming aware of your body and understand when it begins to give unhealthy signs so that you can prevent the injury from happening by taking the proper medications for it.

Before we explore how yoga aids the healing of sports injury, let us quickly identify the injuries that yoga helps to prevent from occurring.

The injuries include:

Hamstring pulls: this is caused by having a tight hamstring and straining of the front or inside muscles of the thigh. This can cause a lot of pain, inflammation, cramps, and even limit mobility, so, it would be better to avoid sustaining this kind of pull.

Hip pain: athletes suffer from an injury because of the quick stop and go movement they experience in sports like soccer and football, they experience hip bursitis, a type of hip pain that occurs in runners and contact sports like ice hockey from pounding the ground, and because of the jarring movements in tennis sports, tennis players are also susceptible to hip pains.

Sprains: occurs when there has been stretching or tearing of the ligament often during a fall. The most common sprain is the ankle sprain which results from an uneven landing from a jump. It is habitual with footballers, soccer players, and track racers.

There are other sprains like knee sprains occurring from pivoting during an athletic activity. Also, the wrist sprain which occurs from landing on an outstretched hand during a fall.

Of course, there are more to sports injuries than what has been mentioned but the focus is on how yoga can help to prevent and hasten sports injury. And without further ado, we would be going into that.

Yoga offers both passive and active stretching poses that can help to both prevent sports injury and under special recommendations by a medical practitioner, hasten healing processes of the sports injuries.

Sports related training can tighten the muscles of the trainer, reduce mobility speed, and even increase chances of incurring injuries during sporting activities. Yoga stretching - both passive and active are very necessary. Basically to allow lissomness in the body tissues and lengthening of the **supta pandagusthasana** muscles to in turn help the sportsperson to become quick in movement and quick recovery from the stress of sports activities.

The sole stretch focuses on the connective tissues and muscles of the sole of the feet and stretches the deep layers of the calf muscles behind the lower leg.

The standing forward bend stretches the hamstring muscles and all of the tissues located at the back of the hips, thigh, and the calf.

The eye of the needle pose also called the *sucirandhrasana* releases tight muscles common in sports that involve a lot of running. These tight muscles can limit movements in the runners and pit more stress in the back of the leg making easy movement almost impossible.

The plank pose, side plank pose, and the cow face pose are yoga practice that helps to relieve shoulder injuries like that rotary cuff inflammation that results from irritation or tearing of the shoulder muscles. The irritation and tearing come as a result of traumatic injury or repetitive motions, especially with an already weak muscle. It is common in swimmers, golf players, and tennis players.

The poses stretch the entire rotator cuff, strengthen the muscles, and stabilize the shoulder blade, which will further contribute to a firm surrounding for the rotator cuff and strengthen their muscles.

Lactic acid build up and yoga

The body prefers to generate energy through aerobic processes but in cases where the body requires energy faster than the body can use oxygen to generate energy, the body does it anaerobically.

Anaerobically would mean generating energy through glycolysis which breaks down the glucose into pyruvate. In cases of strenuous exercise which is common in sports activities, the pyruvate is converted to lactate which allows the breakdown of glucose to energy.

This production of lactate causes the after effects of exercising the body. According to research, the level of muscle soreness after strenuous exercise is determined to an extent by the level of lactate produced by the body during the body exercise or in this case, sporting events.

The lactic acid as a temporary energy source helps you to avoid fatigue during exercise or workout but a build-up would create a burning sensation in the muscles that can rather slow down your athletic abilities.

Now, the way to reduce the production of lactic acids during sports activities through yoga is to start a warm-up with *asanas.*

The *Surya Namaskar* is used as a warm-up before any sports because it moves the spine in different directions and the result is an entire stretched and strengthened body. It would untighten the joints and increase blood and lymphatic circulation in the body. It exercises the cardiovascular system and enhances the regulation of the *pingala nadi* through which oxygen enters the body.

Even though the reduction of the lactic acid build-up through the yoga warm-up practices does not completely eradicate or prevent the delayed-onset of muscle soreness, it is helpful for a much longer and harder workout session which is a beautiful thing for athletes.

Overtraining

If you get into the state of overtraining, you would know because your workout pieces of training will suffer and your performance in whatever sports you do would be affected adversely because the quality you would deliver would be poor. When you notice this, even after doing so many workouts, you would know that you have over trained.

You would feel irritation for the slightest things, get tired from doing very little, become susceptible to injury muscle soreness and you would even become sickly.

The reason is that overtraining triggers a high level of cortisol (the stress hormone) and increases the severity by also lowering the level of testosterone - the hormone that enhances the muscle and strength gain. And together, the over-trainer is both mentally and physically weak for days or even weeks.

Having seen that and you were asked to propose a solution to overtraining, I am pretty sure that you would completely erase more training from your mind and if you do, you would be right. The last thing you want to do in that state is training but to keep you up with a routine, yoga would do the trick.

Yoga might seem similar to exercise but it is not, simply because it is not aimed at building cardiovascular muscles and capacities or even a form of challenge for your body's resistance capacity. Rather, the basic aim of yoga is to help relieve stress and tension. It helps you relax and renew your passion for further exercises.

CHAPTER THREE

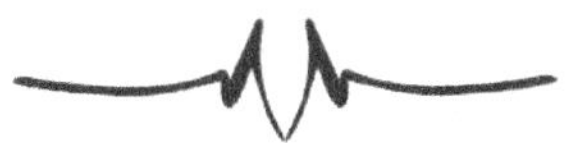

BODY ANATOMY

Football fans are the most energetic and amazing sport fans I have ever come across. Have you ever seen them argue about a game or a favorite footballer or probably been in an argument yourself? Such energy and passion they have for their different clubs and football players.

There are many outstanding footballers in history but one particularly stands out for me; Cristiano Ronaldo of Portugal. I have seen many fans argue for or against him being the greatest footballer of all time but I have never seen anyone argue the fact that he is just different from other strikers; there is something distinctive about him.

You can argue that he is not the best player or argue about the accolades and awards he has gotten in his career but one thing you cannot take away from him is his amazing body and the way he controls it. He is simply a specimen of a perfect athlete; his body makes him special from other football stars. He is still at the top of his game at the age of 34; a point where a lot of top footballers are already past their best.

The amount of time he stays in the air and his abilities to control his neck muscles have been a wonder to the whole world. Sometime ago, after a goal he scored, I saw a paper that read "Ronaldo breaks the law of gravity". I thought to myself, "Ronaldo has mastered anatomy" wouldn't have been a bad headline either.

Thriving in any sports is much more than having the raw talent and skill needed for the sports. The reality is sports has gone beyond that raw talent and focus on improving it. As sports evolved, the science of sports was paid more attention to because the role of science in sports is increasingly becoming very important to the performance of players and teams; athletes need to understand the science of sports if they will ever reach their peak performance.

Athletes need to understand how their bodies work in order to know how to improve their performance and what type of training to pay more attention to for any aspect of their game or skill they want to improve on. The importance of the knowledge of body anatomy for an athlete goes beyond knowing where to improve on and how to improve. It also helps them stay off injuries or recover easily from injuries.

Understanding how the body works

The Golden rule for every design is; "form follows function". Nothing is designed outside of this rule, the human body not exempted. In the context of the human body, this means that every structure in your body is meant to perform a specific and detailed function. The study of these structures and their function is known as anatomy and physiology.

If you want to talk about or understand human anatomy and physiology, you definitely have to start from cells.

You won't even have a body without cells; because your whole body is made up of cells. They are the building blocks of biological life. You have about 37 trillion body cells in your body right now; that's a lot of cells. These cells come together to form body tissues and organ systems which are responsible for specific functions in your body. The cells create four basic types of tissues and eleven organ systems. The integration of the tissues and organ system makes up everything in the human body.

Due to the vastness of human anatomy, we will streamline our study to the major systems in your body that affects sports and performance. We will look at the structure and functions of these key systems and how it affects you as an athlete.

The skeletal system (structure and function)

The skeletal system is largely made up of bones. An adult has about 206 bones running through his cartilage, tendons and ligaments. The skeleton system is basically in the body to give support to all the other systems inside the body. It provides them with a strong framework and structure which protects them. Without the skeletal system, movement and motion will be impossible because it provides the body with structural outline and movement.

The bone provides a lever system against which muscles can pull to create movement, they also provide the joints with fluids that prevents bones from rubbing together thereby reducing friction between the bones. The skeletal system also supports the whole body and carries its weight.

Types of bones

Long bones – long bones are basically the set of bones found in the limbs. They are made up of a shaft called diaphysis; they also have two expanded ends known as the epiphysis. The major functions of long bones are movement, support and red blood cell production.

Short bones – short bones are small light cube-shaped bones made up of cancellous bone surrounded by a thin layer of compound bone. An example of a short bone is the carpals and tarsals of the wrist and ankle. Short bones enable short movements and maintain stability in the body. Its primary function is also to bear weight and act as a shock absorber.

Flat bones – as the name goes, flat bones are actually flat and a little but curvy with a large surface area. An example is the cranium. Flat bones function as protections and attachment for muscles.

Irregular bones – these are bones that have complex shapes which don't fall into any one of those mentioned above already. An example is the spinal column. Irregular bones protect the spinal cord and enables movement too.

Sesamoid bones – these are specialized bones that provide a smooth surface for the tendon to slide over. The largest of them all is the patella which is found in the knee joint. These bones mainly reduce friction and also protects organs in the body.

The human skeleton is divided or spread across two areas or parts namely; the axial and appendicular axis. The appendicular skeleton takes up a higher chunk of bones more than that of axial skeleton; while the axial skeleton is made up of 80 bones, the appendicular skeleton is made up of 126 bones.

However, the axial skeleton is the main core or part of your skeleton and it is made up of:

- The skull (including cranium and facial bones)

- The thoracic cage (sternum and ribs)

- The vertebral column.

The appendicular bones on the other hand, are basically bones that are attached to the axial skeleton, they consist of these parts:

- The upper limbs consist of 60 bones (30 in each arm) including the humerus, radius, ulna, carpals, metacarpals and phalanges. There are a total of 60 bones.

- The lower limbs consist of 60 bones (30 in each leg) including the femur, tibia, fibula, patella, tarsals, metatarsals and phalanges.

- The shoulder girdle consists of four bones – two clavicles and two scapulae – which connect the limbs of the upper body to the thorax.

- The pelvic girdle is also part of the appendicular bones. It is made up of three bones; ilium, pubis, and ischium. They are collectively known as nominate bones. Basically, the pelvic girdle serves the purpose of providing a solid base through which to transmit the weight of the body. It also provides attachment for the powerful muscles of the lower back and legs.

The spine or vertebral column

This is commonly known as the back bone. It starts from the base of the cranium down to the pelvis. The backbone provides a central axis for the body and is made up of 33 irregular bones known as vertebrae. These irregular bones are connected by ligaments which make little movements between adjacent vertebrae possible and also give a degree of flexibility around the spine as a whole.

Joints

A joint is formed where two or more bones meet; this is known as articulation. Joints are classified into three according to the degree of movement possible. The three types of joints are;

Fixed joints – this is also known as fibrous joints. This joint happens where movement is not really needed or desirable although it still gives chance for slight movements e.g. between the radius and ulna above the wrist and the fibula and tibia above the ankle.

Cartilaginous joints - this joint is of two types namely; hyaline and fibro cartilage. The first forms a bar uniting the first rib to the sternum or breastbone while the second is less rigid and allows more movement e.g. intervertebral disc.

Synovial joint – this is the most important joint and the most freely moving joint in your body. The synovial joints are very important to an athlete particularly because it enables you make a lot of movements.

The possible movements in the synovial joint are classified according to their range as it varies in different joints. Athletes use different combinations of joints to make a wide range of movements or perform a technique. For example, a cricketer bowling a ball will need the joints in the finger, wrist, elbow and shoulder to bowl. A sprinter will need the joints in the foot, ankle and hip.

A good coach or athlete monitors the speed of the movements produced by these joints to know where to work on in order to enhance performance.

The skeletal system like any other organ in your body responds to and adapts to physical activity or exercise in different ways. It can give an acute response (immediate response) or long term response to exercise.

Exercises and workouts increase the mineral density in your bone which could lead to having a light weight and stronger bone. It could also lead to more flexibility in your synovial joints especially as a result of increase in the strength of ligaments that attach your bones together to the joints.

Muscular system

The mass of the human body is 40% made up of muscles. There are about 650 muscles in the body. There are also different types of muscle in different places in the human body but once again, lets narrow our study to the skeletal muscle. The skeletal muscle is the most used and exercised muscle in sports because they are the muscles that move our bones and brings about movement and flexibility.

The skeletal muscle is also known as called the stripes muscle because of the stripe-like designs on it. It is an involuntary muscle, in other words, it can be brought under conscious control. Movement happens with the body when the muscle connected to the skeleton through tendons contract, consequently pulling your bones along.

Apart from the skeletal muscle, there are other muscles like cardiac muscle and smooth muscle.

Common skeletal muscles and functions

Hamstrings – the hamstring is located at the back of thigh, its flexes lower leg and extends thigh

Hip flexors – this is located at the lumbar region of the spine to the top of hip joint. As the name goes, this muscle enables flexion of hip joint

Quadriceps – the quadriceps extends lower leg and flexes thigh, it is located in front of the thigh.

Latissimus dorsi – this muscle is large and covers the back of lower ribs. It extends and abducts lower arm.

Obliques – located on the waist, it enables lateral flexion of the trunk.

Gluteal – this is the large muscle in the buttocks, it extends the thigh.

Tibialis anterior – it is located at the front of tibia on the lower leg.

Muscles work in antagonistic pairs; they don't work in isolation. For a movement to happen most of the times, muscles contacts exerting a pulling force on the bones it is attached to. This causes them to move together around the joints. At the point of contraction however, one end of the muscle involved remains stationary while the other part is drawn towards it. Muscles work by pulling and contracting.

There are three types of skeletal muscle contraction namely; isomeric, concentric and eccentric muscles. Isomeric contraction doesn't change the length of a muscle or alters the joint angle. This contraction is very actively engaged when you hold a static position like when you are planking for example during a workout. This type of muscle work is easy to undertake but can easily lead to fatigue.

Concentric muscle contraction on the other hand shortens the muscle as the muscle fibers contract. It is also known as the positive phase of muscle contraction. This contraction is engaged when you make a bicep curl movement for example.

An eccentric muscle contraction happens when a muscle shortens against resistance and then gets back to its normal or original length. This type of contraction is involved in many sports where for example you have to climb, run, jump, etc.

Your muscle also adapts to stress through flexing it while exercising it. It might increase in size due to hypertrophy; become stronger and more flexible when the ligaments and tendons are stretched and strengthened. It can also produce more aerobic energy which leads to better aerobic performance for sportsmen.

The skeletal and muscular system are the most used and important for the performance of athletes, but then other systems of the human body are also quite important. Systems like the respiratory systems, the cardiovascular systems and others, are very important for the wellbeing and stability of athletes. But we can't look at all of them in this chapter due to its vastness.

With the knowledge of anatomy, an athlete can improve the efficiency of his training and perform better.

CHAPTER FOUR

YOGA

Yoga is almost like a household term these days; almost everybody has heard of it. But then, a lot of people still have misconceptions on what Yoga really is. I strongly believe that these misconceptions have their foundation on the fact that the concept of Yoga dates many years back and evolved through ages. It is largely misunderstood in the West especially where it has been confined to physical exercise.

The meaning of yoga goes beyond physical exercise. The word "yoga" is a Sanskrit word which means "union". It is joining two different or separate entities together to become one. Yoga is about unifying our inner nature with that of the universe.

It is one of the six orthodox systems of Indian philosophy. The philosophy of yoga was brought together and systematized by *Pat Anjali* in his classical work, the yoga sutras. The principles of yoga began or started with the Indians but it has spread across the world to the western cultures and like I said it is one of the reasons why it is often misunderstood.

To truly understand what yoga really is about, you have to know the underlying ideology or thought behind its origin and that of course will be seen in the Indian culture and system of thought. In the Indian system of thought, everything is believed to be permeated by the supreme universal spirit (Parramatta or God). Man for example is made of or is a part of the universal force in the vessel of the physical or emotional body which brings different afflictions and experiences to man, but then, the vessel is also a temple through which man can connect with its core; his real self; the universal spirit.

In other words, the human spirit (Jivatma) is a disconnected part of the supreme universal spirit which is the real source of power holding every other thing together. The concept of yoga comes in to unite the separate human spirit to the universal's spirit so as to liberate it from afflictions which come as a result of the disconnection.

Yoga is the art of yoking one's body, mind and soul to the powers of the universe. It is about gaining ascendancy and freeing up one's mind, body and whole being from its restless desires and connecting it to a more powerful force; to God. One becomes one in communion with God by making use of yoga practices to control his mind, intellect and whole being to become absorbed in the spirit within him and overcoming the limitations in his senses.

By overcoming and gaining ascendency over his senses and the limitations around him, such person finds joy and fulfillment and will not be affected by sorrow or trouble. This in fact is the true meaning of yoga; being in unity with the force of the universe and gaining ascendency over the limitations of the senses and sorrows around.

Different Indian gurus have ever since the conception of Yoga, described yoga in their own way but maintaining the central theme or meaning of the concept. The *kathopanishad* for example describes yoga in this manner: 'when the senses are stilled, when the mind is at rest, when the intellect wavers not – then, say the wise is reached to the highest stage. This steady control of the senses and mind has been defined as yoga. He who attains it is free from delusion.'

In yoga sutras, Pat Anjali describes yoga as **'chitta vrtti nirodhah'**. *Nirodhah'* means restraint or suppression, *vrtti* means modifications or fluctuations while *chitta* means mental or consciousness. Putting it together, you would have: "the restraint of mental modifications" or "the suppression of the fluctuation of consciousness". The focus of yoga is to control the mind and make it still from its restlessness and then redirect its energy into other channels free from its restlessness.

The practice of yoga is over a thousand years and has passed through different eras and periods of time in which it continuously evolved and spread across the world. What started initially as more of a spiritual thing is now used in contemporary time by a lot of people as a physical exercise to improve health. This is not to say that it has completely lost its spiritual purpose and function. It rather shows that the practice of yoga has greatly advanced and it is now a practice for all. It fits into different contexts; for sports men and athletes, pregnant women, children, spiritualists, psychologists, etc.

Types of yoga

The spread of yoga which was spearheaded by great Indian yogists like BKS. Iyengar, Swami Shivananda, Shri T. Krishnamacharya, Swami Rama, Shri Yogendara and others has led to rise of different philosophies, practices and traditional schools of yoga. Consequently, there are so many types of yoga and more styles and practices are still emerging today as everybody wants to fit yoga in his or her own context.

Sometimes people new beginners find it difficult to choose a particular type of yoga that would benefit them. The key to choose a type of yoga is to choose what you really want to do instead of looking at what others are doing or want you to do; doing that would defeat the spiritual purpose of yoga itself. The truth is, there is really no right type or wrong type although you might be better off with a certain type of yoga than the other.

I want to help you make the choice of what type of yoga you want to practice, so here is a narrow guide of common types of yoga that you might want to practice:

Kundalini yoga

Yogists have to get use of Sanskrit one way or the other. The word *"Kundalini"* in Sanskrit means "life force energy" which is commonly known as chi or prana in the yoga community. The Kundalini is believed to be tightly coiled to the human spine and is inactive until it is stimulated or unlocked.

The Kundalini practice simply aims at unlocking or stimulating the life force energy of a person and consequently reducing stress and every negative energy within the person. It became popular in the West through the spiritual leader Yogi Bhajan in the late 1960's.

Simply put, the aim of Kundalini yoga is to heighten ones consciousness and make him or her feel great within; unlocking the life force energy. To unlock this force, Kundalini yogists are put through some chanting, singing, meditations and combined poses and breathing work known as kriyas with the aim of permeating and challenging the mind and the body.

In a typical Kundalini Yoga class, the instructor kicks off the class with a mantra which every other activity done in the class should follow. With the class having a focus already, the instructor now put the yogists through some breathing exercise and warm-ups to put the body in motion. Afterwards, more challenging poses are introduced to the class. Then the class is concluded with a series of relaxation and meditation.

This type of yoga would be very fitting for you if you are looking for a combination of physical and spiritual practices and probably with a touch of singing and chanting.

Hatha yoga

The word Hatha is very inclusive; it is used for different schools and types that make use of the body as a means of self-inquiry. However, Hatha yoga got its name from the Sanskrit words for sun and moon. The aim of Hatha yoga is to balance opposing forces. Hatha yoga is often considered to be the traditional physical aspect of yoga. In fact, the balance needed from Hath yoga comes from physical and mental energy, strength and flexibility, or breath and the body.

In a typical Hatha yoga, asana (poses), pranayama (breathing exercises) and meditation must be practiced. Some other types of yoga like Iyengar are also considered Hatha because of their nature. Like I said, it is very inclusive.

In recent times, Hatha is interpreted as slow paced and gentle way of practicing. Beginner yogists are often advice to start from Hatha yoga because it provides a good introduction to the basics of yoga poses in a low-key setting.

This type might be suitable for you if you are looking for a gentler or balanced type of yoga.

Iyengar yoga

A break from Sanskrit interpretation now; Iyengar yoga is named after its founder B.K.S. Iyengar. Iyengar yoga is more known for its constant and effective use of props like chairs, walls, straps, blocks, and bolsters, etc., unlike other types of yoga which considers the use of props optional. Iyengar teachers also undergo through a high level of training.

Iyengar yoga is a classical alignment-based practice which was developed in India and became popular in the

US in the early 1970's. The primary aim is to bring the body into its best possible alignment with the use of props. In an Iyengar yoga class, emphases are placed on holding poses for a longer period of time instead of going through different poses with speed.

Iyengar yoga is perfect for people who like detailed instructions or people with physical disadvantage.

Vinyasa Yoga

Just like Hatha, Vinyasa is a blanket term used to describe a number of practices that is aimed at linking movement with breathing. The word Vinyasa in Sanskrit translates to "place in a special way", hence the interpretation of it as linking breath and movement. This yoga was created from the organized and systematic ashtanga yoga.

Another name for it is flow yoga or Vinyasa flow Vinyasa yoga is a little bit more vigorous style of yoga compared to other styles. It practices a group of poses called sun salutations; every vinyasa class starts with sun salutations and then moves on to other poses. The aim of the glow is to calm the nervous system and mind while in motion. It is very meditative as well.

Anybody can practice this type of yoga though it is especially interesting for those who want more movement and less stillness from yoga.

Ashtanga yoga

Ashtanga yoga is a systematic and organized type of yoga which consists of six series of specific poses that is taught and practiced in order. Ashtanga yogists go through these six series of movement gradually and systematically. They go over to another pose once they have mastered the previous one given to them by their teacher or instructor.

Every pose is personalized and fitted to the growth stage of each student, so in an Ashtanga yoga class, every student has his or her unique move or practice according to the level of growth, allowing students to practice and improve at their own pace.

Ashtanga yoga is a very physical flow style yoga but not totally devoid of spiritual components. Madonna practices this type of yoga in the 90's. One very peculiar thing about this yoga is that no music is allowed in the class.

Ashtanga yoga is very suitable for those that enjoy routines and are also looking for a combination of physical and spiritual practice.

Restorative yoga

I always enjoy seeing the expression of people the first time they come into a restorative yoga class. If you walk into a restorative yoga class, you would be shocked to see that almost everybody is sleeping. Before I go on to explain, if you ever choose this type of yoga don't ever let it replace your good night sleep because it can't really replace it.

Okay, the goal of restorative yoga is to completely relax into poses that would relieve you of stress and down-regulate your nervous system. You are made to relax into poses which can be held for five minutes or more with the help of props to support the body. And you know what; it is very acceptable to sleep off during practice. In fact, sometimes teacher's lead their students through meditations that would place them in-between being asleep and being awake.

Restorative yoga is very suitable for those who find it difficult to relax and for those who just want to relax and relieve stress.

There are so many other types of yoga with slight differences in practice, benefits and purpose. For example, there is the prenatal yoga for expectant women as the name goes. Like I said already, there is something for everyone in yoga, Shivananda yoga, Bikram yoga, power yoga, etc.

Don't wait an extra minute to make the right decision of getting involved in yoga. There are a lot of benefits in yoga which I will discuss in subsequent chapters. But look around you, you would see that a lot of gym centres have adopted yoga practices into their program. In fact a lot of people now practice yoga in their different homes.

You see, you don't have to wait till the right time when you would be free to register with a gym or get a professional instructor to put you through. You can start with the basics anywhere you are and anytime.

CHAPTER FIVE

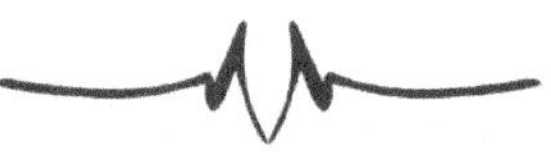

PRACTISING YOGA

In 2016, yoga journal and yoga alliance conducted a study called Yoga America. In the study, they found out that 36.7 million people in America practiced yoga. That was a huge increase from the 20.4 million people that practiced in 2012. The number of people practicing yoga all over the world has remarkably increased over the years. It is predicted that by the end of 2020, over 55 million people all over the world would be actively involved in yoga practice.

The number of people practicing yoga keeps increasing because more people are starting to discover its numerous benefits. Yoga is just the right solution to the modern day or contemporary man whose nerves are constantly stimulated by the numerous activities and complexities in the modern society. Yoga calms those nerves down and restores back peace of mind to the yogists; it creates balance.

There are also the health and physical benefits which we would talk about much more in another chapter. Yoga has numerous physical benefits to keep you fit and healthy; it brings something extra and special to the physical well-being of a sportsperson especially. It is not surprising to see different athletes embracing and practicing yoga these days to increase their flexibility, balance, strength and mobility.

Very importantly, yoga would also relieve you of accumulated stress that would put your system in overdrive, make you feel uneasy, unable to relax or sleep etc. Yoga also benefits yogists spiritually of course by helping them to connect to their sense of purpose and higher self.

These and many more are the reasons behind the increase in the number of people practicing yoga all over the world. It brings a level of upgrade and improvement to anyone that practices it.

Getting started with yoga

The core foundation of the yoga practice was paid in the classic yoga satura by second century sage; Pat Anjali. He introduced and put in place a structure of yoga practice known as the eight limbs of yoga; this is the foundation of all yoga practices.

When a yogist masters or goes through the eight limbs of yoga, he or she is believed to have been able to calm the fluctuations and agitations of the mind to achieve a state of yoga or union also known as samadhi.

Yoga deals with the body, the mind and the whole being of the yogists but it is important to note that yoga practices start from the outward part of one's personality. In other words, the physical body is the place to start with when practicing yoga. This is because when balance is not achieved in the physical body, it becomes difficult for other aspect of the being to align. When the physical body is not balanced, the organs, muscles and nerves no longer function in harmony.

With the help of yoga however, one can solve the problem of imbalance, bringing about harmony and unity in the total being.

The eight limbs of yoga:

- Samadhi

- Dhyana

- Dharana

- Pratayahara

- Pranayama

- Asana

- Niyamas

- Yamas

Yamas

Yama is the first limb of yoga. It is the first of the two limbs that are considered very fundamental in yoga practice. In fact, it is believed that with getting yamas right, other practices would fail to give the desired result. Yama focuses on one's behavior and ethics; it deals with one's integrity and conduct. Have you ever heard of the Golden rule "do unto others what you want them to do to you"? It succinctly describes and depicts what Yama is all about.

There are five Yamas in yoga and they include:

Ahimsa: Non-violence

Satya: Truthfulness

Asteya: Not stealing

Brahmacharya: Continence

Aparigraha: Non-covetousness

Niyamas

This is the second limb of yoga and it is the other half of the two fundamental practices in yoga. Niyamas is like a shade of Yamas, it has to do with self-discipline and spiritual observance. Developing and being consistent with purposeful habits like quiet time and contemplative walk is part of Niyamas. Being regular at spiritual meetings and following their instructions are also part of what Niyamas focuses on.

Just like yamas, there are five niyamas in yoga namely:

Saucha: Cleanliness

Samtosa: Contentment

Tapas: Heat; Spiritual austerities

Svadhyaya: Study of the sacred scriptures and of one's self

Isvara pranidhana: Surrender to God

Asana

This is the most popular and practiced limb of yoga today. This limb deals with postures and placement of the body in yoga. It is traditionally beloved by yogists that the body is the temple of the spirit and the state of the body will affect the rate and efficiency by which one connects to the spirit.

Asana helps yogists to maintain focus or concentration and discipline which helps them to meditate well.

Pranayama

Pranayama, the fourth limb is translated in Sanskrit to mean breath control. It is aimed at controlling the respiratory process while identifying and becoming aware of the connection between the breath, mind and the emotions. Yogists believe that the practice of pranayama extends life just like the meaning of the term itself goes; pranayama means life force extension.

The first four limbs of yoga focuses on fine tuning our personality and integrity, aligning and gaining mastery over our the body and coming to a self-awareness . All these would prepare us for the second stage of yoga practice where we have four more limbs to go.

Pratyahara

Pratyahara means withdrawal or sensory transcendence. In this stage of practice, yogists try to pull themselves out of the external world and their senses and become more connected and conscious of the internal. This however doesn't imply being ignorant of the information in our senses.

The practice of pratyahara enables one to come out of himself and look at his actions and personality objectively like another person would observe. This would allow him deal with some desires and traits that might be a source of imbalance in his being.

Dharana

Dharana means concentration. This practice deals with the mind itself; the pratyahara practice helps you deal with outside distractions and pay more attention to the mind while dharana now deals with the distractions of the mind having successfully become aware of your mind.

The main objective of this practice is to slow down the thinking process and this is done by focusing or concentrating on a single object. The focus could be on the silent repetition of a sound, an awe inspiring image, the image of a deity, a specific energetic center in the body, etc.

The concentration skill you got in the previous stages of practice; posture, breath control and withdrawal of senses would help you do well with this stage. An extended period of concentration would lead to the next limb and level of practice. You would have noticed that the practice of yoga is indeed structural and sequential.

Dhyana

This is the seventh limb of yoga, dhyana translates meditation. Like I mentioned already, it flows from dharana; it is basically an extensive and extended concentration. A lot of people take the two to be the same, yet, there is an important distinctive feature between dharana and dhyana. While dharana is basically a one-pointed attention practice; your attention is merely focused in a single object or direction. Dhyana is the practice of becoming very aware but without focus.

Let me explain further; in dharana you will need to go with your attention on something but in dhyana the mind has been calmed already and in that calmness, it produces very few or no thoughts at all. It takes a lot of strength and process to get to this stage. But don't be discouraged in your journey with yoga because it allows you to progress gradually. And you don't need to perfect each stage to benefit from it; each season or class adds to you hugely.

Samadhi

This is the last limb of yoga. Patanjali described this last stage of practice as the stage of ecstasy. This is the stage where the yogist connects with the force of the universe or the point of focus and transcends beyond his small self to his real self which is part of the energetic force of the universe. At this point the yogist comes to the awareness of his connection with the spiritual real or with divine entities and with that awareness comes the "peace that passeth all understanding".

This might seem unrealistic, lofty and unreal on the surface. But on a closer look at it, you would understand that the experience Patanjali describes here is very realistic, it is what everybody would want to experience.

If you were asked what your goal is in life, I have no doubt that peace of mind would be in your list or at least everything in your list would sum up to having a real peace of mind in this manic world. The final limb or stage of practice in yoga also known as the stage of enlightenment creates an experience of peace and fulfillment not really tied to your physical achievement. It is a worthwhile experience.

The good thing about yoga is; it is easy and flexible to practice. You have the liberty to practice at your convenience, for instance you can decide to register with a studio class/ a yoga instructor or practice on your own; it all depends on what you can deal with at the moment.

If you want to opt for a registered class, you just have to find a practice space that you won't find difficult navigating your way to and make sure they offer classes that fit your schedule and the type of yoga you want to practice. If you want to go virtual, you've got to make sure you would be in the right class or program too.

Common yoga practice settings include; yoga studios around the neighborhood, gyms and athletic clubs, online yoga programs and websites, private yoga instructors and seasonal outdoor yoga events. Some organizations also have an arrangement for work place and corporate yoga.

You just have to make sure you start out consistently with any setting or program of your choice. For example you could decide to practice once or twice a week and stick to that schedule rigidly. Without consistency, you might not see the effect of yoga on you. If you stick with your scheduled practice, it won't take long before you start seeing the effects and benefits of yoga on your body and mind.

A typical yoga class lasts for about 60 to 90 minutes. All through that time, the yoga instructor would teach you and sometimes even demonstrate the poses you have to be on. Towards the end of yoga class, yogists are instructed to lie on their back for several minutes with their eyes closed in a pose called savasana. After the savasana, the yoga teacher says "Namaste"; a word for showing gratitude and thanks which marks the end of the yoga class.

Practicing with a class or an instructor has its advantages and disadvantages too. Some of the advantages of practicing with a studio class are: you will have the support and tutorship of experts to help you develop and improve, you would be more encouraged and boosted when you practice with people and talk with likeminded people in the studio or gym, it is also helpful for a beginner especially who needs to be thoroughly guided into the different poses of yoga.

However don't readily go for studio class sessions because they want or need individualized attention from an instructor which would not be readily gotten in a studio class where there are numerous people practicing at the same time. People like this go for a personalized class/ private instructor or self-practice. Another reason for people not going for studio classes is the cost involved. Studio classes cost more than self-practice or home practice.

A lot of people actually practice at home; some with a private instructor while some practice all by themselves;

according to statistics, 65% of US yogists practice at home. Self-practice especially reduces cost for yogists.

 It also has other advantages; it is more convenient and flexible and also offers you the opportunity to really understand your own body and what you really need. Plus, you don't really have to do it all alone, you can download videos that would guide you or even register with a program online while you practice at home. All you need to do is to create a very convenient space around your home where you would be able to focus.

What it costs?

Here are some stats to ponder on; every year, Americans spend $16 billion total on yoga classes, equipment, clothings, etc. The second stat; an average yoga practitioner spends up to $90 monthly. Last one; in 2015, the yoga industry's US revenue was $ 9.09 billion and it is projected to reach $ 11.6 billion by the end of 2020.

Now the purpose of these stats is to show you how much money that is being invested in yoga over the last few years which of course reflects the value gotten from it as well.

Whether you are into self-practice or registered in a class, yoga would cost you some money one way or the other. At least to buy the equipment and tools you need to start off with and practice. For example, you will need to get items like: yoga pants, tanks, mats, sets of blocks, strap, bolster, etc. And all these would cost money added to the money you might spend if you want to register for any class.

Here's a breakdown for an average class costs:

• Studio package or membership: Approximately $100 to $200 per month.

• Gym membership: Approximately $58 to $100 per month.

• Online yoga membership: Approximately $60 to $150 per year.

• Private session(s): Varies based on the instructor.

Best classes for sports and athletes?

I guess this question have been in your head for some time now as an athlete. So let me just clear you in the type of classes to go for as an athlete to get the most out of yoga and improve your efficiency and performance.

A lot of athletes have practiced yoga to either recover from injury or just to increase their abilities and performance. Professional basketball players such as LeBron James and Kevin Love and American football stars such as Tom Brady and Ray Lewis have practiced yoga. Soccer star and Manchester United legend - Ryan Giggs also practiced yoga during his playing days.

First of all, it is very important you know when to really engage fully in yoga in the long term and short term as well. Because it will determine to a large extent the effect and satisfaction you get from practicing.

You should practice yoga more in your off seasons or break when you are not fully into a competitive season. Because it will avail you the chance to correct muscle imbalances, correct overuse injuries and prepare you mentally for the competitive season ahead of you. It is also advisable to practice yoga more during injuries to help you recover faster and get back to competitions.

This doesn't mean that you shouldn't practice yoga in the middle of intense competitive seasons. It rather means that you have to pay attention to the intensity to which you practice in the different seasons as an athlete. During intense competitive seasons for example, instead of practicing intensively with a style, you can use some poses to just warm up yourself, keep fit before a game or competition and then use it to wind down after a game too. Restorative yoga would also be very helpful to recover and reflect after a competitive game.

Having said that, the best class for an athlete is determined by what the athlete wants - the goal of the athlete. Basically, an athlete might want to practice with the intention of recovering from an injury or gaining back strength while another athlete might want to practice so as to strengthen and improve on some parts of his body or mind. Some might even want to practice for both reasons. So you have got to answer that question; what is your goal for practicing?

Classes are suitable and beneficial to you depending on your goal and the nature of sports you are into. However, there are some classes that don't really fit for an athlete unless recommended by your coach or instructor for definite reasons. Some hot yoga classes like Bikram for example is quite intense and can lead to dehydration which is very bad for an athlete. You might also have to lock your knees many times while practicing and that is not good for an athlete looking to maintain healthy joints.

Powerful classes such as ashtanga yoga, power yoga and vinyasa serve as good cross training for athletes subjected to repetitive muscle patterns at trainings. It is advisable for a runner for example, to practice power yoga in her off day to increase lateral movement and core strength work which will improve her performance on the track.

However, an athlete in the middle of a tight schedule of trainings and works out should practice restorative yoga to calm his nerves and relax a bit e.g. footballers in preseason camp.

Basically all the yoga classes are beneficial for athletes. You just have to know when you should use a class or the other to get the maximum value you need at the moment.

I have heard a lot of people say yoga is for women alone. That is a huge ignorance and misconception on their side and they get to lose for not practicing yoga. The reality is yoga is not gender biased although more women than men are into yoga.

However the rate of men in yoga has been on the increase in the last six years. According to stats the rate of men practicing yoga has increased by 150% in the last four years. The number of yogists in US increased from to 4 to 10 million over the space of 2012 and 2016.

To get the most out of yoga, you have to be consistent because every single minute out into practice would surely improve and benefit you in a tremendous way.

CHAPTER SIX

MOVEMENT

In sports, starting from the basics is something we are constantly taught to do so. The same goes for yoga and movements. It is important that functional movement is learned. Learning movement would help you minimize the chances of getting injuries as you train and also help you maximize the use of your muscles as you move. The role of yoga in enhancing functional movement is extremely beneficial to all professional athletes, a beginner or someone recovering from an injury because it focuses on movement patterns.

There are forms of movement in yoga, the same way other types of physical training have different forms and categories. We would focus on seven forms of movement. These forms of movement are crucial for the health and performance of the athletes.

• Standing Poses – this pose is geared towards building strength in the legs and flexibility in the hips and hamstrings.

• Backward Bends – this improves posture, respiration, digestion, and elimination.

• Forward Bends – this promotes the balance of an autonomic nervous system and the health of posterior chain.

• Balancing poses – this is geared towards increasing body awareness, stabilization, and proprioception.

• Inversions – this improves immune function and enhances circulation in legs.

• Arm Balances – this builds the core and upper-body strength and improves body-awareness.

• Twists – this improves posture, shoulder-mobility, respiration, digestion, and health of spine and nervous system.

Importance of movement for sports

Core strength: these movements train your core to keep your spine stable through various movements. It is important to remember that every form of exercise and yoga involves our core, so these movements imitate the demands our core makes on our spine regularly.

Posture: working on posture can be tasking. If you have had someone who worked on their posture or if you have had to, you would know that it isn't the easiest thing to do. Functional movement can help correct bad posture and any other effect from stress, daily activities or even poor exercising techniques that may cause certain imbalances in the muscle.

Balance: functional movements enhance stability and improve balance. How this works is that the movement focuses on certain muscles that enhance stabilization.

Joint mobility: functional movement training can enhance the mobility of your joints. This improvement stands out more when one is going through the recovery process (from an injury or from surgery). It can also improve your motion generally.

Muscle tone: there is usually an upgrade in the balance between one's body weight and the movement of the muscles. Functional movement creates a tandem between the two, channeling the body weight to control the muscles and the motions as seamless as possible. This movement strengthens and also tones the muscles.

Preventing injuries: taking part in sporting activities without having the right movements can leave you dealing with injuries. It is imperative that you learn simple movements before applying the pressure that comes from sports on your muscles. Having the right movement is one of the best ways to prevent injuries.

Tracking movement using Fitbits and app

The amount of technological devices made over the years for tracking movement has evolved continually from being able to track steps to tracking heart rate and cholesterol. In the last three year Fitbit movement tracking devices have been made with an improvement that included yoga. These movement trackers have been planted as chips in yoga mats made into watches, headbands and implanted in other devices. This new innovation has helped a large number of people monitor their movement and keep their bodies and health in check. Experts have emphasized the importance of moving and exercising your muscles for a few hours daily.

The common yardstick is taking 10000 steps a day and the lifelong benefits it offers an individual. Imagine you had to track how many steps you take every day without the help of all these technological innovations that have been made available. How would you successfully determine how many steps you have taken per day?

One of the most common movement trackers is the fitbit. It is worn on the wrist by many. It tracks steps, sleep cycles, heart rate, and many other things. The big question is how does fitbit do this? It has been shown that the fitbit tracker can count steps accurately. How it does that is the million dollar question? Fitbits can interpret a number of your movements. They can tell when you're simply walking, jumping, running, or tapping away on a table. They can do this by using the three-axis accelerometer, which can correctly determine if a person is moving backward, forward, to their side and back or up and down. Determining these movements allows the fitbit to tell what activity you are engaged in, whether it is walking, running or jumping.

Fitbits runs by several algorithms that work together to correctly determine your positions or the movements you're making. It can tell if you're not in motion, if you're moving speedily, if you're moving on one foot or both feet, or when you're in a vehicle or when you're moving parts of your body like your arms. The data it provides on your steps can be trusted because it rules out through the algorithm those movements that weren't steps and counts the actual steps you took.

Counting your steps on a Fitbit

To see the total steps you took at the end of the day:

- Press the main button on the side of the fitbit.

- either tap the screen to view different stats or push the button on the side several times.

Or

- Open your fitbit app on your phone

- Go to activities and click "today"

Or

- Go to your dashboard on your computer

- Go to activities and click "today"

Benefit of keeping your joints moving

Many of us sometimes forget that we would be immobile without joints. Movement is impossible without joints. Human joints are of varying shapes of size and are responsible for a number of our regular activities. On certain occasions, our joints are sometimes injured as a result of different reasons. These injuries may lead to a series of discomfort and pain. Statistics show that a good number of hospital visits associated with pain are joint related. The joints in the knee, ankles and shoulders are the commonly injured joints.

The joints in the body consist of two surfaces or more touching each other. These touching surfaces allow for easy movement because joints are made to withstand pressure and allow for seamless movement. Types of joints are: hinge joints (elbow and knee), gliding and sliding joints (spine), ball and socket joint (hip). The muscles in the joints are responsible for the production of movement while the bones allow this movement to happen.

For joints to work, they need strong tendons to aid movement. Tendons are what join the muscles to bones. Tendons are flexible enough to prevent muscles' tissues from getting damaged and strong enough to aid movement. The tendons don't work alone; they are backed-up by ligaments. Ligaments connect bones, they are stiff and prevent the joints from moving unaided and excessively. These three (ligaments, tendons, and muscles) work together. They are found in specific parts of every joint. Friction between these attachees is prevented by the fluids in the joints which lubricate the joints and allow the joints to be used for a very long time.

Moving your joints is important for its lifelong functions. The joints do not receive blood like the other parts of the body, therefore our daily movement is important for the health of our joints. The movement of our joint is as important as every other aspect of joint maintenance and care. Lack of use does not do your joints any good. Movement is vital for the health of your joints. Here is why: a good number if not all the joints in your body are lined with cartilage. A cartilage is a firm and flexible tissue that is found on the surface of joints. These cartilages are nourished by a process called imbibition which involves pushing the synovial fluid into the cartilage. The entry of the fluid into the cartilage occurs through pressure within the joints and the only way this pressure occurs is when the joint is moving. When bones move against each other without a cartilage, it can lead to the tearing up of bones, bone spurs, degenerative joint diseases and many other joint diseases.

Still on the importance of moving your joints, the human spinal disc consists of the annulus fibroses and nucleus pulpous. The annulus fibroses is the outermost and larger of the two parts of the disc; it is like a ligament. The nucleus pulpous is the inner gelatinous part of the disc. These two parts of the spinal disc also get nourished by the imbibition process, which also means they are fluid-based and require movement for this nourishment to happen. For the gliding joints in the spine to be fully functional, movement is imperative.

Movements coupled with good dieting would help your joint function and prevent joint wear and tear. A generally healthy living would help your joints stay healthy and attain its long life expectancy.

CHAPTER SEVEN

MOBILITY

Mobility is often confused for flexibility, but they actually do vary and hence we have it that while flexibility is the ability for the joints to move without restrictions and pain through a range of motion, mobility is the strength of the muscles in that range of motion. To show flexibility, they would be needed for assistance, like being able to move your leg or your arm further with the help of the other arm. But mobility is being able to move the leg only with the muscles of the leg.

Mobility is necessary for stress training; exercises that train the body's mobility are done to properly prepare the body for the stress they have to undergo during workout training.

According to researches, Mobility is essential for minimizing the risk of injuries during training and actual sports activities.

Having a good mobility helps the body communicate to the brain when an injury is about to happen because it helps to eradicate pain and aches from the body. With a good mobility, you move pain-free in the gym, in your sport field, and in your day to day routine.

You would not have issues stretching to pick up stuff from your high shelves or pick up something from the ground when it drops.

And as you age, it is advisable you maintain good mobility training to enable free movement all over the place because with aging come restrictions in the joints and easy mobility is affected.

The question now might be how exactly?

The answer to that is that good mobility helps the joints to heal and regenerate with the endogenous energy and lubrication it provides.

The athlete ought to train for mobility and the reason is that, during mobility training, blood is sent to the surrounding tissues in the body and the fluids that help the joints to slide softly and freely are transported to the joints that perform the exercises.

For example, during mobility trainings, the synovial fluid helps the hips to glide freely during the actual workout and athlete.

This is the reason why Mobility is said to resume the risk of injury, once there are no restrictions of movement in the joint areas, there is a very low risk of incurring joint related injuries.

Of course, different sports come with varying flexibility demands from the athlete to avoid injuries.

With Mobility, training comes with flexible joints and muscles and this results in a larger range of movements and the result of this is better performance at sports and easy adaptation to a better technique of training as they come.

Athletes depend highly on their bodies for competitive games and sports to enable them to be better than their opponents and without good mobility, the body is unable to get them the win.

Without mobility, the body of the athlete will break down and athletic abilities will be lost. You want efficiency in sporting performance and high flexibility of the muscles and joints, your mobility must be up in the game. The athlete or just anybody must pay attention to the capacity of the shoulder, neck, hips, knees, ankles, and back and wrist movements if they intend to be proficient in their line of sports.

Every time a basketball player runs or jumps, they extend in their ankles, hips, and their knees, throughout a game, to shoot a ball and defend an opponent, their ankles, hips, and knee joints glide, and when they have to squat through a game, they use their hamstrings, calves several other thigh muscles of which with low mobility their performance would be affected adversely. With all the movements they have to move at different joints and with different muscles, both in the back, shoulder, thigh, arm, and chest, it is very important that basketball players require high mobility capacity to ensure eminent performance in their sporting competitions. Because definitely, if any of the joints (ankle hip, knee) are unable to make full range motion, the player would perform poorly and incur injuries for attempting full range motion with their tight joints.

Lastly, a limited range of motion would mean limited growth of muscles. It has been proven that mobility training enables the sportspersons to improve their knee extensions, flexion, and more thigh muscles. This in turn boosts their capabilities of which you can translate to strength. Better mobility is better strength; it means faster and more efficient.

Think yoga, think flexibility, think better mobility.

The *budokon* yoga can help the body improve in the mobility and flexibility of the joints. It combines mobility, flexibility, strength, stamina, and endurance because, in actual sense, it is a combination of yoga, martial arts, dance, and animal locomotion.

Several other yoga moves help the athletes reach optimum levels that concern mobility, some of which are;

Acroyoga: also called the inside flow. They say that this is where you would likely experience the limitations of your mobility and flexibility capacities.

Child pose: important for relieving tension in the spine and neck and increasing the space between the shoulders and the vertebrae.

The cat-cow: also releases tension in the neck and spine and promotes flexibility.

The cobra yoga: helps to stretch and strengthen the back, the chest, and the shoulders. It strengthens the spine and stimulates the internal organs for better performance.

Warrior one and two stretches Thames shoulder, chest, thigh calves, and ankles. They strengthen the arms and legs and tone them as well for endurance.

CHAPTER EIGHT

LONGEVITY

I would simply buttress my point by giving you reasons why yoga would improve longevity;

Balance

Yoga practices improve body balances and proprioception. Balance is both coordination of the physical being and the symmetrical balance of the body from left to right, front to back, and up to down. Aging comes with the loss of balance but with yoga practices, it can be delayed and the aging man or woman can still move about agile. Yoga achieves through its breathing and physical exercises that help to strengthen the core of the body and improve reflexes. The strengthening of the core and improved reflexes is how the body can balance physically and hormonally.

Heart attack

Yoga practices boost heart rate aerobically. It assists the body to take in more oxygen and cause the heart rate to increase and this lowers the risk of a heart attack. It helps the mind get rid of depression and stress which can cause a heart attack. And more to it, yoga helps the body to lower blood pressure, reduce blood sugar and cholesterol. All these of course can improve the wellbeing of a person and increase longevity.

Joint breakdown

This is one of the most important reasons athletes need yoga, and as they age, it can help prevent cases like degenerative arthritis because yoga prevents the wearing and tearing of joints by providing them with nutrients. And with a wider range of motion it provides, the underlying bones in the joint areas are protected and arthritic cases are greatly prevented.

The asanas help to strengthen the muscles so that there is less strain on the joints because weaker muscles would drive the body to rely on the joints for stability and this could cause a breakdown.

Yoga moves allow the circulation of synovial fluids in the moveable joints and this would mean that the bones at the joints area would glide freely without grinding.

Deeper sleep

From living in such a busy and mind-boggling era, the nervous system of our body needs some soothing. And yoga and meditation can provide this soothing optimally by stimulating deeper and sometimes longer sleep, to mean less feeling of stress and fatigue all over the place.

Survey shows that over 60% of people that practice yoga slept better and 80% were relieved of the stress feeling they had. Balasana is a resting pose that provides a sense of calmness.

Digestion

Yoga poses and practices promote healthy digestion of food. Certain yoga movements facilitate the easy transportation of food and elimination of waste products through the canal and this has helped to reduce the chances of colon cancer and any diseases of the digestive tract.

The answer to uneasiness after having too much to eat or feeling of stomach rumbling because of indigestion is not always unbuttoning your clothes. Yoga provides you with better chances of gaining a long-lasting relief instead of something ephemeral.

Yoga aids digestion and waste eliminating, even bloating by increasing circulation and energy channeled to the alimentary canal. Yoga calms the sympathetic nervous system to decrease stress and tension and in turn, activates the parasympathetic nervous system for easy digestion. It stimulates the internal organs to promote harmony and balance which also helps for easy digestion and release form body wastes and bloating.

For self-care

The truth about staying consistent with yoga practices is that it helps your mind in vast ways. Yoga by itself has the power to inspire the stimulation of good hormones in the body that cause you to feel good and inspire you to do more. It inspires you to take care of yourself and live healthily primarily because of how good it makes you feel even after only a few practices. So you become more aware of what routines to follow and ensure that you stay healthy and lively, and if this wouldn't promise longevity, I do not know what else will.

The breathing practices boost the immunity system against cold and flu. Yoga helps the body find relief from inflammations even the chronic inflammations.

These and much more are the reasons why yoga practices can be very beneficial for ensuring longevity. Who wouldn't be happy to thank themselves later in life for the freedom of joint movement win old age, for maintaining healthy habits and suffering from no heart attacks or hormonal imbalances that are common with aging because they invested their time practicing yoga?

And, the beautiful thing is that it can be practiced by all age groups even though you would better do yoga as a young male or female when you have all the strength you can get in your lifetime. Investing your time and energy in yoga practices now would save you from physiotherapy bills and the disability that comes with old age.

So, there's more to it, aside from ensuring longevity, it allows to age strong. Compared to your contemporaries, you would be doing a lot better as you age because you would have more strength and stay straight longer than the normal age.

Trust me when I say that flexibility and good mobility in old age is a beautiful thing to behold, much more than that, to have.

CHAPTER NINE

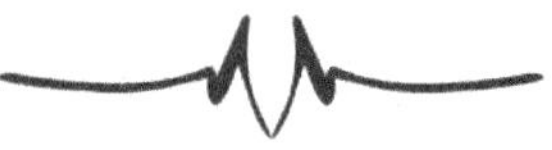

LIFELONG BENEFITS

The concept of yoga originated in ancient Indian philosophy. There are different types of yoga (Viniyoga, Iyengar, Sivananda and so). Every one of them has their distinct emphasis from breathing to postures, to meditation and relaxation practices. The application of yoga as a therapeutic practice started in the 20th century and it maximizes all the benefits of the individual types of yoga. This benefits the general wellbeing of the yogist. For example, the physical exercise- asanas would most likely increase strength, flexibility, and balance. While the breathing and meditation enhances focus and reduces anxiety.

The sporting benefits of yoga goes beyond just physical effects, it also affects the mental health of athletes. Unlike other forms of exercise, the effects of yoga are usually lifelong, working for both young and old. It is a lifelong and life-enhancing practice that brings lifelong results.

The big question is, does Yoga truly lead to a better sporting life? Yes it does- both physically and mentally. Athletes who have yoga practices incorporated in their training have experienced benefits of yoga that goes beyond just being flexible.

Here is how yoga helps you mentally:

● Reduces Anxiety: Anxiety is a real thing for competitive athletes because of the environment they have to perform in. The pressure to perform and win is always present especially in sports where money and their reputation are at stake. The constant pressure can lead to anxiety and tiredness, mentally. It is exerting to be under pressure physically and also mentally. Finding ways to deal with both external and internal pressure would definitely help to improve performance. Yoga is that way. Athletes who practice yoga have been shown to be more relaxed and less mentally tired. The reduced anxiety or the ability to control anxiety they develop from their yoga practices helps them improve their performances.

● Mental Fortitude: Endurance/fortitude is more mental than physical. The ability to hold out in an uncomfortable physical situation many times has more to do with mental fortitude than physical might. There are poses in yoga that involve holding a position/pose for a period. At this time, muscles are tested as you try to maintain balance and hold the pose at the same time. This helps your endurance levels. We are constantly told to build mental fortitude and yoga is how it is done. It helps you push and hold out.

● Mental Focus: Athletes are continually trying to push themselves physically. This is important but those who truly stand out are the ones who build mental strength. Yoga helps athletes stay focused even through uncomfortable positions because it sharpens the mind.

Athletes are encouraged to try out pregame yoga, because it lets them focus and improves their breathing.

• Perceiving Sensation: Physical improvement differs from physical perception. It is the difference between getting more flexible and knowing the feeling of being more flexible. Yoga allows you the opportunity to pay attention to your body and everything you feel. This is crucial for an athlete's increased performance. The athletes that practice yoga get to explore and experience their own physical limitations and can make the best decisions for their bodies based on the feedback they receive from their bodies. Understanding sensations and learning how to make positive decisions based on this feedback is a skill that helps the athlete gain and exercise control over how they perform and their bodies in general.

• Proprioception: this is the ability to perceive stimuli arising from the body regarding position, motion, and equilibrium. Through yoga, you get to experience your body in fresh and amazing ways. Familiarizing yourself with your body's ever changing position in space is crucial and vital in advancing performance in athletics. This ability to control the body and adapt fully to external changes beyond our senses expands our likelihood to compete more mentally than physically.

Regularly practicing yoga can have the following physical benefits

• Injury prevention: Injury during sports or training can slow down an athlete's performance. Yoga improves your body's awareness and mechanics there by reducing the chances of getting injuries during sporting activities or during training. This benefit allows athletes to progress through the course of their careers injury-free, many times.

• Improved Recovery: Yoga enhances circulation and lymphatic flow, which is one way to get improved recovery. The benefits of yoga go beyond enhancing strength and endurance to speeding up the body' metabolic rate, thus increasing the body's healing and recovery time

• Increased Power: Most athletes know that power, strength, and speed are all connected to their proper body mechanics. A properly aligned body can transmit force efficiently and improve the general performance of the body. Whatever the form of sport, by returning your body to its peak alignment, yoga helps you reduce wastage of power in your dead cells, improves running posture and efficiency, and makes you fit for whatever sport you're involved in.

• Better Endurance: Yoga significantly increases respiratory capacity. There are testimonies of individuals who have overcome respiratory conditions, like asthma, through constant practice. Postures in yoga enhance breathing. Yoga has also been proven to speedily improve digestion, circulation, and efficiency of motion, which greatly improves energy and endurance.

• Proprioception: Yoga builds greater body awareness and opens the body. It gives balance, stability, and proprioception. This increases efficiency in training and enhances our performance.

Other lifelong benefits of Yoga

● Cardiovascular Benefit: There are athletes who have to deal with cardiovascular issues like hypertension and strokes as they get older. Heart issues stem from a combination of different things. The most common being: poor lifestyle choices, poor dieting and negative thinking and emotions. These things basically stir up a chain of unhealthy chemical reactions, which tells the body that something is wrong. Yoga helps the athlete breath and take in enough oxygen.

● Back pain: Back pains usually come from tension in the muscles that support the spinal cord and stress. It is easy for athletes to get back aches especially from the tension at the spinal cords. Other causes may include bad posture issues that have lasted for a long time unattended. Yoga reduces back pain issues by allowing the circulation of blood and balance. It also helps to prevent future back injuries that may arise.

● Managing Pain: Yoga is said to reduce pain by helping the brain's pain center regulate the gate controlling mechanism located in the spinal cord and the secretion of natural painkillers in the body. Breathing exercises used in yoga can also reduce pain. Because muscles tend to relax when you exhale, lengthening the time of exhalation can help produce relaxation and reduce tension. Awareness of breathing helps to achieve calmer, slower respiration and aid in relaxation and pain management

• Respiratory benefits: Practices of Yoga (Asanas) have helped reduce cases of Asthma and other respiratory problems. When the nasal passages get inflamed, they start producing mucous in excess, making it difficult to breathe and often have common symptoms like coughing, wheezing etc. Respiratory problems could also be caused by multiple factors like allergy, exercise, weather change, etc. By practicing yoga, the lungs capacities increase and so does stamina and stress on air passages reduce.

Other benefits include;

• Stable autonomic nervous system equilibrium, with a tendency toward parasympathetic nervous system dominance rather than the usual stress – induced sympathetic nervous system dominance.

• Pulse rate decreases.

• Endurance increases

• Energy level increases

• Endocrine function normalizes

• Excretory functions improve

• Cardiovascular efficiency increases

• Respiratory efficiency increases (respiratory smoothness increases, tidal volume increases, vital capacity increases, breath –holding time increases).

- Galvanic Skin Response increases

- Respiratory rate decreases

- Muscular-skeletal flexibility and joint range of motion Increases

- Posture improves

- Strength and resiliency increase

- Blood pressure decreases

- EEG-alpha waves increase (theta, delta and beta waves Also increase during various stages of meditation)

- Gastrointestinal function normalizes

- Weight normalizes

- Sleep improves

- Immunity increases

- Pain decreases

- Yoga improves and strengthens deep connective tissue thereby preventing or minimizing injury.

- Creates an overall body flexibility.

- Increases range of motion and mobility.

- Enhances physical balance by developing the athlete's awareness of his body's center place, thus keeping their body balanced in action, giving the ability to recover from or prevent falls, while enhancing agility.

●   Improves circulation, massages internal organs and glands for optimum health.

●   The yoga breathing process allows circulation and detoxifies the lymph fluids to speed up recovery time from training 15% faster, eliminating fatigue.

●   The yoga breath builds up and increases one's life force energy.

●   Enhances sensory acuity, mental focus, concentration, mental clarity, will power, and determination.

●   Dissolves pre-competition anxiety and stress. Helps to balance & manage emotions that could cloud focus, concentration & judgment.

CONCLUSION

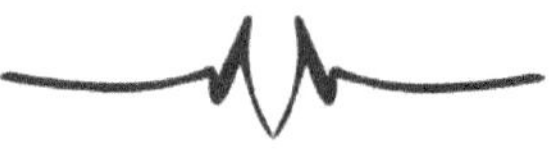

Yoga for athletes is a tool to improve and transform their performance. The lifelong gains of yoga for an athlete cannot be overemphasized. The distinctness of the effect it has on the physical aspects of an athlete is transforming when compared to any other forms of exercise. Yoga practices are not supposed to replace the regular training; the goal is incorporating yoga into regular training to improve it. Every form of sport: soccer, basketball, American football, golf, cricket and so on, can benefit greatly from yoga. Putting it simply, Yoga is what differentiates the strong, flexible and balanced athlete from other athletes.

The benefits which have been explained thoroughly during the course of this book are encompassing. They cover the physical, the physiological, and the psychophysical aspects of a person. By contributing to building mental fortitude, yoga helps the athlete endure and improve performance because many times, the difference between the successful athlete and others is their mental strength. Building core strength, posture, enhancing balance, toning muscles and preventing injuries are key ways to improve an athlete's performance. Yoga practices in sport training are gaining popularity fast; the positive and lifelong effects are encouraging more people to participate.

The spine and its components can be considered as one of the most important physical attributes humans have aside from the brain. This is because every move the body makes originates from signals sent from the brain through the spinal column. All our body parts connect to the spine in one way or another. Other physical training methods barely focus on the spine. Yoga turns this around by focusing first on the spine because if the spine is in order, other parts of the body would benefit strongly from it. In yoga, it is the spine before other body parts. Athletes learn how to use their spine properly during the yoga process and come to an understanding of the different areas of the spine function. This is an effective secret weapon that many athletes have honed through yoga while they unlock other lifelong healthy movement patterns.

The focus of this book has been on making lifelong benefits from this life changing activity called Yoga. It is important that athletes remember that improved performance in sport is possible and not just possible for a short period but for the long run even when they are old and can't fully participate in whatever sports they are doing now. Incorporating yoga into your daily sport training would bring a transformation to your physical health and your mental health likewise. Don't cheat yourself out of this great opportunity to enjoy and perform greatly at your sport.